Yin Yoga for beginners

Gentle exercises and simple asanas for less stress, more relaxation and holistic health - including a tried-and-tested example sequence

Mira Steen

⚡ CONTENTS

What you can expect in this book

Relaxing baths, reading books, calming teas, lavender, walks, breathing deeply: do these aids sound familiar to you in your search for more inner balance and on the path to greater equilibrium? Are you often easily irritable in everyday life and wish you could react more calmly to many situations? Do you often lie in bed at night and wonder when you will finally be able to calm down and fall asleep? Then this guide may be able to help you. It deals intensively with a type of yoga that calms the body and mind and allows the soul to relax. Yin yoga - a contrast to the often hectic pace of everyday life, which is dominated by yang. Try it out and find your own daily ritual that you can always look forward to and which is not only good for your body's health, but also brings the peace and inner harmony that so many people long for these days.

Let's discover the benefits of yin yoga together and delve deeper into the subject matter. Understand the background and apply the practice immediately at home, so that from the first contact with this way of letting go, you can be more at one with yourself again and thus face life's small and big adventures with more self-love and contentment. Take a deep breath - and let's go!

A little theory is a must

YOGA - WHAT IS IT ACTUALLY?

Describing the history, forms and trends of yoga in general would certainly fill several books in itself, but ask yourself this simple question: how would you explain to someone in just a few words what yoga is? It's not that easy, even though the word has become an integral part of health and lifestyle. Yoga is an ancient (approx. 3000-4000 years) philosophical teaching and originates from India. The roots of yoga philosophy lie in Hinduism and partly also in Buddhism. The aim is to bring body and mind into harmony.

This is not only encouraged by numerous different physical activities, but also supported by various breathing exercises and meditations. Yoga teaches you to accept yourself, to be completely with yourself and to experience self-love, harmony and happiness. The aim is also to reduce stress, recharge your batteries and practice mindfulness and self-awareness. Over 300 million people worldwide practise this spiritual sport and yoga was even recognized as an intangible world cultural heritage in 2016. There are around 130 different types of yoga and the field is constantly evolving. In the following, however, we will only focus on one type of yoga, one of the gentlest variants, which is also very suitable for an introduction to the world of yoga - yin yoga.

ORIGIN OF YIN YOGA

This special type of yoga has its roots in the 1980s. Yin Yoga was developed by the American Paulie Zink from various other types of yoga, such as Hatha Yoga and Tao Yoga, and further developed by his student, Paul Grilley, and his student, Sarah Powers. The latter also gave Yin Yoga its name.

Y IN AND YANG - MEANING

Yin and yang, black and white, the description of two opposites that everyone has heard of. The black and white circular symbol, which looks like two intertwined tears, comes to mind. These each have an oppositely colored dot in the middle. In Chinese philosophy, this explains the two complementary streams of life, the two complementary energies. Yang - the bright, active, moving, day, sun. Yin - the dark, passive, calm, night, moon. This pairing of opposites could be continued endlessly. What is striking, however, is that they are always components that are not completely mutually exclusive but, on the contrary, are mutually dependent. In other words, one would not exist without the other. Both are needed for balance and equilibrium. This symbolism can also be applied to the human body and mind. On the one hand, body regions can be divided into yin and yang areas. For example, the lungs, heart, liver, kidneys and everything inside the body belong to the yin area, while the bladder, intestines, gallbladder and the outer layers of the body, including the skin, belong to the yang area. Traditional Chinese Medicine (TCM) uses this classification to explain the structure and also pathological changes and their healing and the physiological functions of the human body. However, this topic would go too far here and should not be considered further.

However, a distinction can also be made between more yin and more yang activities in terms of physical activity. Harmony and balance of both forces are the goals of various yoga practices. Yang is trained through dynamic, more muscle-focused exercises (Ashtanga yoga, for example), while yin is characterized by staying in certain postures for a longer period of time. In yin yoga, the muscles are used less and the exercises are performed more in conjunction with gravity and stretching of the fascia and tendons. Balance is the magic word.

"Yin yoga is necessary to bring our yang-heavy culture into balance."
Paul Grilley (founder of Yin Yoga)

WHY YIN YOGA?

In this day and age, there are as many sport and activity options as there are excuses not to get started with them. But why should you choose yin yoga of all things? Because it's somehow "in", i.e. trendy, or because you want to have a say if the topic comes up at a party or among colleagues?

These are certainly not reasons that lead to a long-term and sustainable practice of Yin Yoga. But ask yourself, what can I do for ME? What is good for me, my body and my mind? How can I reduce stress (and let's be honest, everyone can list a number of stressors in their life off the top of their head, no matter how different or supposedly inconsequential they are)? Or: How can I manage to be more balanced and less irritable? Do the questions sound like this or something similar in your head more and more often? Then it is quite certain that practicing Yin Yoga will help you.

The motivation should therefore come from within. You have to make the decision yourself to want to change something and become active for your own improved well-being. The aim is to increase your own quality of life and to benefit to a certain extent from the serenity and balance you have gained in your everyday life.

You are the focus here. Yin yoga is a slow form of yoga with asanas (postures) in which you spend a long time, usually sitting or lying down. This allows you to feel your own body and come to rest. The nervous system is automatically calmed and you feel calm, balanced and relaxed after a yin yoga session. It is therefore beneficial for the soul and mind. However, regular practice also has other physical benefits, such as increased flexibility and stronger muscles. You have probably also heard of fascia training. Fascia is the name given to the deeper layers of connective tissue in the body. They envelop all muscles, bones, tendons and organs and are of great importance for posture and stability as well as supporting muscular work.

Lack of exercise, stress or overloading can cause the fascia to harden, stick together or twist, which can lead to various types of pain. Yin yoga addresses precisely this elastic connective tissue, allowing it to relax and do its actual job again. If these aren't all reasons to start this wonderful form of yoga very soon!

FOR WHOM IS YIN YOGA SUITABLE?

As Yin Yoga is less dynamic, as already described, and jerky movements are completely avoided, this practice carries little risk of injury. It can therefore also be practiced by people who may have an increased risk of injury in other sports or who may already have physical limitations. Individual exercises for certain areas of the body can simply be skipped or replaced with similar asanas. In addition, the necessary equipment is limited to a few items, which will be discussed later. There is no need for expensive purchases or courses, which can sometimes diminish the desire for the new activity or even put you off completely before you start.

Experience in other types of yoga is certainly an advantage, but not necessary, as the individual asanas are explained to you in detail so that you can also practise yin yoga at home on your own on the yoga mat. The overall concept of Yin Yoga also offers a welcome addition and a great balance for enthusiasts of other sports, which can presumably be classified as Yang (dynamic, more active).

Similar to the effect of a fascia roll, practising yin yoga stimulates the connective tissue and loosens any adhesions, for example due to sitting for too long or a lack of movement. If you have joint or spinal complaints, please consult your doctor about which movements you should refrain from or which exercises may be particularly good for providing you with relief.

This also applies to women during pregnancy. However, the respective exercises can always be adapted to individual circumstances and needs. You can also decide for yourself at any time how intensive you want the exercises to be and carefully discover the limits of your own body. Regardless of whether your goals are to improve your physical fitness or flexibility, to gain new energy and mental abilities or to relax and reduce stress, by practising Yin Yoga regularly you will always come closer to achieving them.

Overall, yin yoga is therefore suitable for anyone who wants to regain their inner balance and do something good for their body and mind. But be careful - the gentlest type of yoga definitely carries a certain risk of addiction!

WHAT DO YOU NEED FOR YIN YOGA?

First of all, you need to feel completely comfortable. This means wearing comfortable trousers and a top that is not too tight. Your clothes should allow you to move freely and warm your body at the same time. As Yin Yoga is mainly practiced sitting or lying down and therefore involves little strenuous movement, you can also put on warm woollen socks or cuffs, for example.

We also recommend the so-called onion look, i.e. several layers on top of each other, so you have the option of taking your clothes off or putting them on again depending on the intensity of the exercise. Place a softer yoga mat underneath so as not to jeopardize your relaxation on the cold, hard floor.

However, a carpet could also be enough for you to try out the exercises for the first time. If necessary, aids such as yoga blocks and yoga straps can also be used. These are essentially there to reduce the distance to the floor if you are initially immobile or to make the exercises easier. However, they are not absolutely necessary to start with Yin Yoga. A simple sofa cushion or a folded blanket have exactly the same benefit. Similarly, external feel-good factors such as scented candles, incense sticks, a delicious favorite tea before or after the Yin Yoga sequence and calm music are not absolutely necessary, but can significantly help you to calm down and switch off during the exercises.

Simply try out what you like best over time, or vary according to your mood and mood of the day. However, an important prerequisite for this is a quiet environment. This can be a place in your home or, in the warmer months of the year, a place by the lake, in the garden or wherever else you simply feel good. In addition, a blanket can provide you with cozy warmth during the final relaxation or be placed under your knees during individual exercises to make the position more comfortable.

So you see - in principle, it is possible to try out the exercises of Yin Yoga just like that and at no extra cost. The market for beautiful yoga accessories is large and you can gradually find your favorite pieces, or you may prefer to be purist and concentrate on the essentials and create the necessary environment with items that you already have in your household. The choice is yours - and as always, balance is the key: Balance is the key.

W E APPROACH THE PRACTICE

So, when are we finally going to start the exercises? A little patience - before we actually get on the mat, you should understand what is really important in Yin Yoga. You should fully engage with the exercises. It will certainly be a little unfamiliar at first. Sporting activities are more often associated with the idea of movement and exertion than with staying in a posture and coming to rest, and then mainly sitting or lying down. But you will be rewarded for your curiosity about something new with an extraordinary grounding, the feeling of living more consciously in your body again and also showing it gratitude. Immerse yourself in the wonderful world of Yin Yoga.

Y in yoga - let's go!

"Yoga is 99 percent practice and 1 percent theory."

We will now follow this quote from Sri Krishna Pattabhi Jois, an Indian yogi, by getting on the mat together.

THE E INDIVIDUAL ASANAS

There are 25 different asanas, i.e. postures of the body, in yin yoga. As these are held for between three and five minutes, only a few of them are selected and practiced in a yin yoga session instead of a long series of exercises in succession. Of course, it depends on how much time you have and how long you want your training to be, there are no limits.

In the following, the asanas are presented individually and their execution is clearly explained as well as the positive effects on body and mind. After each asana, a balancing pose is also described, which you should assume after releasing the pose in order to relieve the region of the body that has just been stressed and to feel the exercise performed. In this way, the body achieves balance and gradually learns to cope better in this posture the more often you do these exercises and their compensation.

The second-mentioned terms after the common German names are the original Sanskrit names of the corresponding asanas, which are also often used by the teacher in yoga classes. In preparation, place any aids you may have within easy reach and make sure that you are not disturbed from outside (loud noises, draughts etc.) during your yoga practice. Then take your time settling into the different postures and gradually come to rest. Breathe in deeply through your nose and either exhale through your nose with pleasure or exhale through your mouth with an audible sigh. Don't worry about how you look or sound during the exercises, but focus solely on yourself and your body.

Arrive at the asanas and feel how your different body regions feel, which exercises you may already find easy or where regular practice is needed. Every body is different and comparisons are out of place here. Every day is also different and practising in the morning can feel more cumbersome than training in the evening, when you have already done a lot of exercise in your everyday life, because your tendons and fasciae are still shortened from sleeping. Do what works best for you intuitively. If you ever have the feeling that you can no longer stay in one position, do yourself a favor and release it.

The yoga practice should offer you added value and it is extremely important to listen to your own body and not exceed its limits. You can also close your eyes from time to time to fully listen to yourself. Give yourself a moment of mindfulness. Yin yoga is not just a sporting activity, it should touch you in a deeper, spiritual and grounding way.

1. the seated butterfly - Baddha Konasana

The pose called butterfly is a gentle hip opener. These are often found in yin yoga. Physically, they are intended to improve your mobility in the hip joints and contribute to a healthy posture. Emotionally, in this pose you can let go of everything, check off the past and simply let your feelings take over.

Execution

Sit on your yoga mat and bring the soles of your feet together in front of you. How close you place your feet together from your buttocks is up to your body and how you feel. Now relax your knees and let them fall gently towards the floor, supported by gravity. Then lean your upper body forward and allow your back to round. (Note: unlike other types of yoga, where a straight back and a tense posture are important, in Yin Yoga you can completely relax your muscles and not exert any strength or effort in the exercises). Your hands now either clasp your feet or lie on the floor in front of you. The palms face upwards. Experienced yogis and yoginis can already place their forearms and head on the mat here. Don't worry if there is still too much distance here. One way to relieve the strain on your neck is to take a blanket or similar and place it on your feet or legs and rest your head on it. Now stay in this asana for three to five minutes. Simply let your thoughts pass and relax every single muscle.

Equalizing posture

After you have slowly released the posture, place you both legs on the mat in a sitting position and let your knees sink alternately to the right and left towards the floor. This movement is often jokingly referred to as a windshield wiper. Mobilize your hips and feel the stretch you have just performed. You can place your hands behind you to take some of the strain off your back.

Positive effects

If you practise the seated butterfly regularly, you will gain flexibility in your hip joints and even the cross-legged pose, which is probably a little difficult at first, will become a relaxed posture in which you can meditate, for example. The lower back and hamstrings also experience a pleasant stretch in this asana. This exercise is beneficial for bladder problems and is good for the kidneys. Mentally, this pose stands for lightness and beauty, also similar to a butterfly.

2. reclining butterfly - Supta Baddha Konasana
A variation of the sitting butterfly is the lying butterfly. To do this, lie on your back. Bend both legs and let your knees sink outwards. Now let the soles of your feet touch each other. As with the butterfly, the distance between your feet and buttocks is again up to you. Just as it feels good for you. If this is too much of a stretch for you at the beginning, you can take two blocks or cushions and place them under your knees or outer thighs. Place your hands comfortably on your lower abdomen and feel the slow rise and fall of your abdominal wall as you inhale and exhale deeply and with pleasure. Your head rests heavily on the floor during the exercise. Your eyes are closed. Remain in this pose for approx. three to five minutes. Allow your breathing to flow and surrender to the gentle stretching of the hip joints and groin. The balancing pose and the positive effects are similar to the seated butterfly and have already been described above.

3. the child's pose - Balasana
Execution

The starting position for this exercise is sitting on your heels. The knees are mat-width apart and the big toes are touching. The backs of your feet are flat on the mat. Now walk forward with both hands, keeping your buttocks on your heels. If you have sensitive knees, you can use a woollen blanket as a support. Place your forehead on the mat and transfer your body weight to the mat. Your back is now completely long and all tension can be released.

As a variation, take both arms back and place them close to your body. The palms of your hands should be facing upwards. The shoulders can sink down quite heavily here, while the shoulder blades fall apart. Your forehead also rests on the mat and you simply release all your muscles. This variation is a little more passive than the child's pose described above, as you can also influence the stretching of the shoulders by stretching and slightly rotating the arms.

Equalizing posture

As a simple balancing pose, lie on your back and stretch your legs out in front of you. Feel the regions of your body that you have just worked on and stay in this position until you are ready for the next yin yoga exercise.

Positive effects

Your shoulders are gently stretched here and the lower and middle back can also be prepared and warmed up for more difficult backbends thanks to the pleasant stretch. This asana also calms the heart, helps to relieve tiredness and headaches and you will find peace and quiet almost naturally.

4. the Sphinx - Ardha Bhujangasana (and the Seal)

Execution

Lie in a prone position for this exercise. Raise one leg at a time and pull it straight back, then put it back down straight. Support yourself on your forearms, which should be pointing forwards. Your palms are resting on the mat and your fingers are spread wide apart. The middle fingers point forwards towards the short end of the mat. The elbows are placed directly under the shoulders, which tend to be pulled back.

Keep your legs together and press the backs of your feet gently into the floor. Keep your head in line with your spine to relieve pressure on your neck. Stay in this position and make sure that your lower back does not tense up. The buttocks remain loose and are not tensed.

In this pose, however, activate your center and press your pubic bone lightly onto the mat. If you like, you can also practise this exercise a little more dynamically. To do this, lift your upper body slightly higher as you inhale. Stay like this for a short moment and lower your body again as you exhale. Repeat this sequence around five times. For a more intensive version of the sphinx, push your hands further forward and lean on both hands to create a stronger backbend and more intensive stretching of the entire front. Here you should pay particular attention to the lower back, as it is under extreme strain. Incidentally, this pose is now called the seal.

Equalizing posture

The child's posture, as described above, offers a wonderful balance here. Apply pressure to your hands lying on the mat. Take your time, as the lower back first needs to get used to this counter movement.

Positive effects

This asana helps with tension in the upper back. However, as there is also a lot of pressure on the abdomen, women should avoid this pose during pregnancy. The entire front of the body is stretched here and the muscles of the back and buttocks are strengthened. Sphinx opens your heart, gives you self-confidence and also relieves anxiety.

5. the happy baby - Ananda Balasana
Execution

For this further hip opener, which is often referred to as a happy baby, lie on your back and bend your legs. Now grasp the outer edges of your feet with your hands from the inside. The soles of your feet should point towards the ceiling and your legs should be at a ninety-degree angle. The shins are in a vertical position. The knees point towards the mat and the lower back rests completely on the mat. The shoulders are relaxed and also rest on the mat. The neck remains long and the head is laid back. Now gently push your feet into your hands and, in contrast, pull your legs down slightly with your hands to create a good balance.

Equalizing posture

After three to five minutes, simply lie on your back and feel the exercise.

Positive effects

Here, the hips are stretched intensively, while at the same time calming the mind and counteracting stress and fatigue. In this pose, the image of a happy baby actually comes to mind, beaming at you in this pose and making this exercise look child's play.

6. the dragon - Anjaneyasana
Execution

Dragon is one of the most active poses in yin yoga. To perform it correctly, start by standing on four feet. Now bring your right foot forward between your hands. The right knee is above your foot and does not point forward beyond the ankle joint. The back left knee moves a little further back and you place it back on the mat. Make sure that there is not too much weight on the left knee. You can also place a blanket underneath to protect the knee. Put your back foot over so that the instep rests on the mat. Now slowly and carefully lower your pelvis down and experience a stretch in the leg that was placed backwards. You can keep your hands on the mat or lean on your right knee. You can leave your head in line with your spine or lower it slightly downwards. Stay here for three to five minutes and then change sides.

Variants of the kite

Assume the position as described above, but now place both hands on the inside of the front foot. You can also bring it a little closer to the outer edge of the mat and place it on the outer edge and push your knee out slightly. If you want more, rest on your forearms. In addition to stretching, this also opens up the hips and the position is a little more intense. Another variation is the twisted dragon. To do this, keep your hand on the side of the leg that is stretched back on the mat and place the other hand on the knee that is on the same side. Now open your upper body to the side of the raised leg and choose your own intensity of the twist by pressing your hand on the knee or front thigh. You can also increase the intensity by releasing your hand from your knee and stretching it vertically upwards. You can return to the starting position at any time.

Equalizing posture

Here too, the child's posture is an ideal compensation posture. You can adopt this both after the exercise and before changing sides.

Positive effects

This asana can have a beneficial effect on sciatica. It also opens up the hip area and groin and stretches the back leg and front thigh muscles. It is also intended to release all tension and provide an overall balance to our mostly sedentary everyday activities.

7. the caterpillar - Paschimottanasana
Execution

This exercise starts in a seated position and is also called a seated forward bend. Stretch both legs forward
and make sure that you are sitting firmly on the mat
on both ischial tuberosities. To do this, you can use y-
our hands to lift each half of your buttocks backwards
once. If it is uncomfortable or too strenuous for you, sit
on an elevation, a yoga cushion or a rolled-up woollen
blanket. Now bend your knees slightly and round your
back forwards. To make the position more comfortable, you can also place a blanket under your knees
and rest your head on a vertical or horizontal yoga
block. You do not need to actively pull your body forward with your hands, but can let gravity take its
effect. The leg muscles are always relaxed. Your hands
lie loosely next to your legs. Your palms are facing the
ceiling. Let your shoulders sink down in a relaxed position.

Equalizing posture

Place your feet on the mat for a counter movement and
place your hands on the floor behind you. Then move
both knees alternately to the right and left on the mat
again.

Positive effects

The caterpillar gently stretches the entire spine, which benefits your entire posture.

8. the (sleeping) swan - Rajakapotasana
Execution

To perform the swan pose, also known as the pigeon pose, stand on four feet. Now place your right foot between your hands. Move your foot slightly further to the left and gently place your knee and lower leg on the floor to the right. Now stretch your left leg backwards and place it completely on the floor. The back of your foot touches the floor. Now lean on your forearms, which you place on the mat in front of your right knee, and bend your entire upper body towards the floor.

For the sleeping swan variation, place both arms on the floor and also bring your forehead to the floor. If you decide to do this variation, first return to the forearms when you release the asana, stay here for a few breaths and then release the pose.

Equalizing posture

As a balancing pose, stand on your four feet and move your spine alternately into cow and cat pose. To assume the cow pose, assume a slightly hollow back and raise your gaze slightly forwards. Open your thoracic vertebrae and heart. For the cat, make the familiar cat hump and round your back as much as possible. Feel your belly button pull inwards and upwards. Perform this dynamic exercise slowly at your own pace and in a controlled manner. You can also practise this counter movement before changing sides.

Positive effects

This asana stretches the hip flexor, which is neglected by a predominantly seated posture in everyday life.

9. the snail - the plow - Halasana
Execution

Start this exercise lying down and place a cushion under your buttocks. Now lift your legs upwards into an inverted position. Initially, keep your arms next to your body with your palms facing upwards, then bring your legs over your upper body and your feet over your head. Now bring the cushion further under your back with your hands and place it back on top. You can open and bend your legs slightly. You can now hold your feet with your hands or interlock them at the back of your knees. Gravity will now do the rest and you can indulge in the stretch.

Breathe into the stretch in your lower back and relax your shoulders. As a variation, you can go further into the plow pose. To do this, bring your legs even further back so that your feet touch the floor or a cushion positioned there. You can use your hands to support your lower back here. Drop your knees down towards your ears. Stay here for approx. three to five minutes and come out of the exercise mindfully.

Equalizing posture

Lie flat on the mat and stretch out your legs. Stretch both arms backwards and place them on the floor. Take a few deep breaths and feel the scroll or plow exercise.

Positive effects

This pose stretches the leg muscles, the internal organs are massaged by the compression and the blood flow to the heart is stimulated. Any blockages in the spine are released and the exercise has a harmonizing effect on the thyroid gland.

10. the saddle - Supta Vajrasana
Execution

Start this exercise in a quadruped position. Now open your lower legs slightly wider than hip-width and carefully lower yourself backwards. This exercise is very intense for your knees and thighs. If you notice a pulling sensation, place a blanket on the mat on which you are sitting down. Then bring your arms behind your back and support yourself on the floor as you slowly and carefully lie backwards. You can also use cushions or blankets to reduce the distance to the floor to make it easier to lie down.

One variation of the saddle is the half saddle. To do this, extend one leg forwards and then lie backwards. After remaining in this position, change the side of the outstretched leg as a matter of course.

Equalizing posture

For balance, lie on your back without any cushions and place your feet on the floor. Again, move both knees alternately to the left and right in synchronization. Enjoy the release of this intense posture and feel for yourself.

Positive effects

The saddle opens up the lumbar spine and stretches the hip flexors and thigh muscles. This pose is particularly good for people who stand and walk a lot in everyday life.

11. the deer - Jathara Parivartanasana
Execution

Sit on the mat with your feet in front of you. Now lower both knees to the right. Position your right shin so that it is parallel to the front edge of the mat. The left leg is bent backwards. Now turn to the right with your spine stretched upwards. Your left hand holds your right knee and your right hand is placed loosely on the floor behind your back. Each time you inhale, you become a little taller and straighten up further. With each exhalation, turn a little further to the right. The chin remains above the sternum the entire time and is not turned in further than the upper body.

This asana can also be intensified. To do this, place your upper body on the mat or on a folded woollen blanket to the right. Also place your forehead on the floor. You can also increase the stretch here by taking the back leg further back.

Equalizing posture

We also recommend alternating the rotation of the knees, i.e. the windshield wipers, while you are sitting on the mat and your feet and hands are positioned.

Positive effects

The rotation of the upper body aids digestion and this position is also said to alleviate general menopausal symptoms.

12. the banana - Bananasana
Execution

Lie on your back and stretch your legs out on the mat. Take both hands behind you and stretch them out as well. Now walk your entire body with your legs closed close to the right edge of the mat. Now move your upper body and both arms to the left so that your body takes on the shape of a half moon or banana on the mat. Then grasp your right wrist with your left hand to stretch even more in a controlled manner. Now breathe into the right side of your body, which will experience a pleasant stretch. After about three to five minutes, change sides.

Equalizing posture

Before changing sides and after the exercise, simply lie straight on your back for a few breaths and feel the twist and stretch.

Positive effects

The banana, also known as the half moon when standing, opens the lateral fascia connections and has an extremely calming and balancing effect.

13. the eye of the needle - Sucirandhrasana
Execution

This asana also begins in a supine position. Place both feet on the floor. Now place your right ankle on your left knee. Then grasp your left thigh with both hands and gently pull it towards you. The right arm reaches here as if through the eye of a needle, hence the name of this pose. If you have lifted your upper body to grasp the thigh, slowly lower it back to the floor. Here too, you can control the intensity yourself by pulling your left thigh more or less towards your sternum. You can also use your right arm to push your right knee further outwards, away from you. If you are very practiced in this position and want more, you can also grasp the right shin instead of the thigh. Remain in this position for three to five minutes and then switch sides.

Equalizing posture

Again, remain lying straight on the mat before changing sides and after the exercise. You can also stretch your arms behind your head and stretch or put your feet up for a short moment and raise your hips to form a bridge. Move your body intuitively and do what feels good for you.

Positive effects

The eye of the needle stretches the hips and gluteal muscles.

14. the shoelace - Gomukhasana
Execution

Get into a quadruped position. From there, place your right knee between your two hands on the mat. Now sling your left leg over your right leg. Now open both lower legs and place your buttocks on the floor between your lower legs. Now bend your entire upper body forward and rest it on your legs. Round your back and let your head hang relaxed. Place your hands on the mat in front of your legs. As a variation, you can also place your hands on your knees and rest your forehead on your hands or on an additional cushion or woollen blanket. Remain in this position for approx. three to five minutes, come into the balancing position and then change sides.

Equalizing posture

As a simple balancing pose for the asana known as cow face in other types of yoga, lie flat on your back and feel the intense stretch.

Positive effects

This pose activates the lateral gluteal muscles and relaxes the region of the lower back. It also stimulates the internal organs - gall bladder, liver and kidneys.

15. the frog - Bhekasana
Execution

To perform this asana, place a woollen blanket folded lengthwise across the mat to cushion your knees. Then get into a quadruped position and slide your knees as far apart as possible on the blanket. At the same time, stretch your arms forward along the floor. Start by keeping your feet together and your buttocks between your legs. As soon as you feel the stretch in your inner thighs, you can move your feet further apart. Now lower your upper body a little further down and find yourself in the intense frog pose.

Equalizing posture

Here, the child's posture is the counter movement. The legs are closed here, so bring the knees back towards each other. Feel the position of the frog and take a few deep breaths.

Positive effects

This asana is an intense opening of the inside of the legs and can help to harmonize emotional and impulsive moods. It also stimulates the stomach, spleen and kidneys.

16. the toe sit - Vadrasana
Execution

The starting position is again the quadruped position. Place the toes of both feet on the floor and slowly begin to straighten your upper body in order to carefully sit on your heels with your buttocks. This unaccustomed stretching in the toes can be quite intense. Only go as far as you can hold for a few minutes.

Equalizing posture

Lift your buttocks up and gradually tip your toes over again so that the backs of your feet are flat on the mat. Now slowly sit back down on your heels. Doesn't that feel very good? Feel the asana you have just performed for a few breaths.

Positive effects

A number of fasciae converge in the feet, which are stimulated by this pose. The feet and toes are also loosened and, according to the followers of Tao Yoga, "a person with open toes also has an open mind".

17. the dragonfly - Upavishta Konasana
Execution

This posture begins in the sitting position. Place a folded blanket under your buttocks again so that you can sit up straighter. Then straddle your legs as far as possible and bend your upper body forward. If the stretch is not enough for you, first try to place your forearms parallel to the front and then possibly even your forehead on the floor.

As a variation, you can also practice the dragonfly on the wall. To do this, you need a wall surface that is not quite so cold and wide enough to stretch your legs out on. Place the yoga mat lengthwise against the wall at a right angle. This means that the short side of the yoga mat is against the wall. Now sit sideways against the wall and lie on your back. Then bring your legs up against the wall and move your buttocks all the way up against the wall. Keep your feet closed and align y-our body once again in a straight line. Rest your arms comfortably on the floor or on your lower stomach.

As you exhale, simply stretch your legs apart and let them slide down along the wall. Do this slowly and carefully. Now relax in the position you can stay in for longer and breathe deeply into this hip opener. Stay here for a total of three to five minutes and notice that your straddle becomes deeper and deeper on its own over time. Recharge your batteries with this exercise and take your time to release the position.

Equalizing posture

Follow this wonderful exercise in a simple supine position for a few breaths. After the dragonfly on the wall, you can also put your feet up and let your knees sink alternately to the left and right. This small mobilization of the hip joints should be performed gently, as the straddle is an intensive stretch.

Positive effects

The dragonfly opens the hips and groin and stretches the inner thighs. It stimulates the liver, kidneys and bladder and releases a lot of energy.

18. the heart opener - Anahatasana
Execution

Start in a quadruped position. Stretch your arms forward and place both palms on the floor. Then lower your upper body down and rest your forehead on the mat. Keep your hips above your knees. If you cannot reach the floor with your forehead, you can place it on the palms of your hands placed on top of each other or on your stacked fists. This will reduce the distance to the floor again. Get into a position that is comfortable and feasible for you and stay there for three to five minutes. Take deep breaths and lower your upper body a little further with each exhalation. For a twisted version of the heart opener, stretch your right arm forward and thread your left arm far under your right armpit. Then place your left arm on the floor, palm facing upwards, and your head on your left temple on the mat.

Equalizing posture

Before changing sides and after the exercise, it is best to adopt the child's posture to compensate. To do this, place your arms back next to your body with your palms facing upwards. The back can round here and

make a counter movement to the exercise just performed.

Positive effects

The heart opener stretches the shoulders and has a balancing effect on the heart area. It is a gentle backbend
for the middle and lower back and warms up gently.

19. the (supported) shoulder bridge - Setu Bandha Sarvangasana
Execution

Start this asana lying on your back. Place your feet hip-width apart on the mat. Bring your heels as close to your buttocks as possible. The arms are at the side of the body. Press your feet firmly into the floor and slowly lift your pelvis. Roll upwards vertebra by vertebra. You can stay here and keep your pelvis as high as possible. At the same time, press your arms into the floor. However, the knees should not be kept apart, but rather held together energetically.

As a variation, cross your hands under your buttocks and stretch your arms forward. Pull your shoulder blades together and jerk your arms closer together so that you are resting on your shoulders instead of your entire back. Meanwhile, always keep your pelvis in the highest position. Your buttocks remain relaxed and your neck long. Stay here for three to five minutes and then lift your heels off the floor and roll back down onto the mat, vertebra by vertebra.

Equalizing posture
To balance, lie on your back and feel the previous stretch for a few breaths.

Positive effects

The entire front of your body is stretched and the spine becomes more flexible. This wonderful backbend opens the heart and acts as an effective mood enhancer by stretching the thoracic spine and ribcage.

20 The Camel - Ustrasana
Execution

Kneel on your mat for the camel pose. The upper and lower legs are closed and the feet are touching each other. The backs of your feet are flat on the mat. Now place your palms on your sacrum and push your hips forward. Protect your lower back by tensing your abdominal muscles. With each inhalation, stretch the length of your spine and with each exhalation, gently lean your upper body backwards to open up the thoracic vertebrae. As soon as you are able to do this stretch, place your hands on your heels one after the other. To make the stretch easier and shorter, you can put your toes up so that they are easier to reach with your hands. The head remains in line with the spine and is not overstretched backwards.

Equalizing posture

As a counter-movement, lie on your back and bend both legs. Grasp your knees with both hands and rock gently on your lower back from side to side or make small circular movements, then change the direction of rotation.

Positive effects

As a version of the backbend, the camel stretches and strengthens the spine and back muscles, which can alleviate and prevent back pain. This very opening position also releases tension, stimulates the abdominal organs and reduces stress.

21 Cat's Tail - Marjarasana
Execution

Start here by lying on your right side. You can rest y-our head in the hand of your right arm or on your upper arm. Whatever is most comfortable for you. Bring your left leg forward and place it on the mat at an angle. Bend your right leg backwards and grasp your right foot with your left hand. Then push your left shoulder back a little further so that you come into a comfortable twist. Now stay in the gentle twist of the cat tail for three to five minutes.

Equalizing posture

Before changing sides and after the exercise, stretch y-our arms and legs out for a long time to bring your spine back into alignment. Feel for yourself and take a few deep breaths.

Positive effects

This asana stretches the front thigh muscles and the hip flexors and is therefore a good counter-movement for bending forward or a predominantly seated posture in everyday life.

22. the square - Samachaturasana

Execution

For the square pose, sit in a cross-legged position that is comfortable for you. Your feet can lie on top of each other or behind each other on the mat. Now stretch upwards and lengthen your spine. Now walk forward on the mat with both hands and place your forearms parallel to each other. If possible, rest your forehead on the mat or on a cushion. Keep your back straight during the exercise.

Equalizing posture

As a counter-movement, lie on your back and place your feet on the floor. Now lower both knees alternately to the left and right side. This mobilizes the hip joint and brings it back into balance.

Positive effects

The square stretches your entire back and shoulder area. It opens the hips and groin and gives you new energy.

23 Squat - Malasana
Execution

This asana begins exceptionally in a standing position. Open your feet hip-width apart, with your toes pointing slightly outwards and your heels pointing more inwards. Now bend your knees to come into a squat position. If you lift your heels off the floor here, you can place a blanket under them for support. Now place both hands in prayer position in front of your heart, i.e. palms facing each other and fingertips pointing upwards, and gently press your elbows against your inner thighs. This allows you to determine the intensity yourself and adjust it to your needs during the exercise. Now lift your chest up and pull your shoulders back so that your back is straight. This allows you to enjoy the width in the front of your upper body and remain in the squat position for three to five minutes.

Equalizing posture

To compensate for this hip opener, lie on your back and place your feet mat-width apart. Now let both knees fall towards each other in an X-shape and take a few deep breaths.

Positive effects

This pose strengthens your front shin muscles and o-
pens up the hip and groin area. This improves your balance and Malasana also has a stabilizing and calming
effect on the mind.

24 The Crocodile - Makarasana
Execution

Start this pose lying on your back. Place your arms flat and stretched out on the floor at right angles to your body at shoulder height. The palms of your hands touch the floor. Now place both feet on the mat and let both legs sink to the right. The legs remain closed here. Try to keep both your left shoulder and right knee on the floor. To intensify the twist, look to the left towards your left hand. In this pose, pay attention to your lower back, which receives special attention here. Remain in this asana for three to five minutes and take a few deep breaths.

As a variation, you can now also stretch out the leg on top to increase the stretch. The exercise can also be adapted by placing your opposite hand on the leg or knee and either letting gravity alone help or gently pushing it towards the floor.

Equalizing posture

Stretch out both legs and place your arms close to your body. Feel the twist in the simple supine position and then change sides. This exercise is often followed by the final resting pose, Shavasana, to end the yoga practice.

Positive effects

This exercise, which is an intensive twisting exercise, stimulates detoxification of the body. It also releases tension and keeps the spine flexible. This asana calms the nervous system and is often performed towards the end of a yin yoga session to bring it to a gentle conclusion. Stress is reduced and peace and strength can enter the mind.

25 The back relaxation pose - Shavasana

Yogis and yoginis end each of their yoga sessions with this asana, which literally translates from Sanskrit as death pose. It is therefore not a pure yin yoga pose, but rather a common final pose in all types of yoga to end the yoga practice. In this final relaxation, the energy that has been activated by the previous exercises is distributed throughout the body and it comes to a final rest and a state of absolute relaxation.

Execution

You lie on your back in Shavasana. To stretch your lower back, first place both feet on the mat. Now lift your buttocks briefly and move them as far as possible towards your feet to put them down again.

The lumbar spine has now reached its maximum length. Then place both legs on the floor again, about as wide as a mat. Lift your legs up one after the other for a moment and stretch them away from you, heel first, then put them down again. Let your feet fall loosely outwards. To open your chest, pull your shoulder blades towards each other once and then relax your entire shoulder area.

Also stretch your arms towards your feet one after the other and place them not too close, but next to your body. The palms of your hands should be facing upwards. Now turn your head slowly and carefully from left to right and from right to left a few times. When you have leveled it back in the middle and lifted your chin slightly towards your chest to lengthen your neck, your entire spine is in a line on the floor. If you have problems with your lower back, you can place your feet as wide as a mat and let your knees fall towards each other in an X-shape.

This description is quite long for the fact that you end up just "lying on your back", but the conscious and correct positioning of the individual body parts is relevant and supports this posture, through which you will achieve pure relaxation.

Now let go of everything. Close your eyes. With each breath, release more weight onto the floor and feel heavier and heavier. Feel your body touching the floor with the largest possible surface area and grounding you on the mat. Then let your breath flow and come and go naturally without thinking about it. Likewise, your thoughts simply pass by and all pressure and tension fall away from you. You can stay in this wonderful pose for up to ten minutes. If you feel that you want to come out of Shavasana, do so gently. Start by consciously breathing in and out deeply again. Start to move your fingers and hands, toes and feet.

Make circular movements and finally stretch your arms and legs and stretch out. Everything is allowed here and you make the movements that intuitively feel good to you. Then come into a seated position - preferably with your eyes closed - preferably sitting cross-legged.

Once again, powerfully raise both arms up over your sides. Bring your palms together above your head and assume this prayer pose in front of your heart. Thank yourself and your body for this wonderful yoga practice you have just completed and feel the energy in your body, mind and soul.

YIN YOGA FLOW

A yoga sequence is usually divided into three phases. It begins with a brief arrival on the mat. This means that you lay out your yoga mat and any tools you may need within easy reach and eliminate any external distractions. Then sit cross-legged and bring both hands forcefully up over your sides.

Breathe in deeply and bring your hands down in front of your heart in a prayer position as you breathe out. This could be a great way to start a yoga session and allows you to focus on yourself and your body. Alternatively, start by blocking out the stress of everyday life by lying on your back for a few minutes and closing your eyes.

This is followed by the main part, in which certain asanas are practiced. The sequence is up to you or can be taken from a predetermined plan. This part takes up most of the time, but does not always have to take up to an hour to be successful. Even a few exercises and a shorter practice time have an effect, especially on balance, because you have actively taken time just for yourself. Yin yoga sessions can also last up to two hours because, as you have experienced, the individual asanas are held for a few minutes and a balancing pose in between also takes time. You are therefore free to organize your time as you wish and can flexibly carry out your yoga practice every day. At the end, the final relaxation, Shavasana, brings you to complete relaxation and distributes the spiritual and physical energy gained from the asanas throughout your body. You will be guided back into everyday life and end your yoga practice for today. Here's to welcoming your mat back soon!

EXAMPLE OF A YIN YOGA SEQUENCE AND HABIT

The following is an example of a complete yoga sequence.

Now that you have become familiar with the various asanas of yin yoga, here is a possible yin yoga flow, i.e. a sequence of asanas that can be practiced one after the other. Basically, the individual asanas are building blocks that can form a yoga unit in any order. As they address and stimulate different regions of the body and also have different effects on the mind, you can choose them depending on the situation and your current mood or which area of your body needs a little more attention at the moment. You can also find this out by practicing mindfulness in general and listening to your body. It is best to read through the sequence of asanas and then look back at how to perform them correctly in order to get the best possible results and deepest relaxation from this yin yoga sequence. Then take your time and bring the tools you need within easy reach and arrive on the mat. Then start practicing the asanas in sequence.

Yin yoga sequence:

1. The heart opener
2. The deer (right and left)
3. The dragonfly
4. The dragon (right and left)
5. The banana (right and left)
6. The Sphinx
7. The posture of the child
8. Shavasana

Afterwards, thank yourself for taking the time to do something good for your body and mind. How was it - your first yin yoga practice? Isn't it wonderfully grounding and energizing at the same time to pay so much attention to your body and to stretch and feel areas that are often neglected in everyday life? How about a daily habit? Depending on how your daily routine is structured, you can start a regular yin yoga practice in the morning after getting up or in the evening before going to bed or even as a lunch break in your home office, which - according to scientific studies - will become a habit after 66 days at the latest. You will probably even miss something if you don't have time or don't feel like moving on the yoga mat.

Everything is one - and the one is eternal

Yoga as a spiritual immersion in the self. Arrive completely with yourself. Being in the moment. Blocking out everything around you and focusing on your own body, mind and soul. Sounds too good to be true or to become true? However, this state can be learned. By practicing Yin Yoga regularly, you can get a lot closer to it and if you commit to it, you can even achieve it. Everything is one - and the one is eternal. These words are intended to motivate you to practise various asanas and thus to create your own personal yin yoga session. At the beginning of your yoga practice, it may of course be that the yoga asanas described above cannot all be performed perfectly immediately or that the desire to engage in physical activity quickly disappears. But remember: no master has yet fallen from the sky.

This requires patience and serenity as well as the will to do something good for yourself. Take time for yourself and your body and you will quickly discover the positive effect that practicing yoga has on your everyday life.

Simply let go of the outside world for the time you need and focus on yourself and within yourself. This will help you to relax and reduce the stress and worries that surround you.

You are welcome to continue accepting and practicing the aids listed at the beginning, such as relaxing baths, reading books, calming teas, lavender, walks and breathing deeply. Breathing deeply in particular is very similar to practicing Yin Yoga. However, you will no longer need it entirely to calm down and ground your mind, as this will happen automatically as a positive side effect once you get into a regular yoga practice.

Strength lies in tranquillity. Give yourself time to immerse yourself in this new world and feel the success in your own body and mind.

With this in mind: stay relaxed at all times.

www.ingramcontent.com/pod-product-compliance
Lightning Source LLC
Chambersburg PA
CBHW021132130726
47988CB00003B/1265